NO AR

SO-AEE-018

Health Care

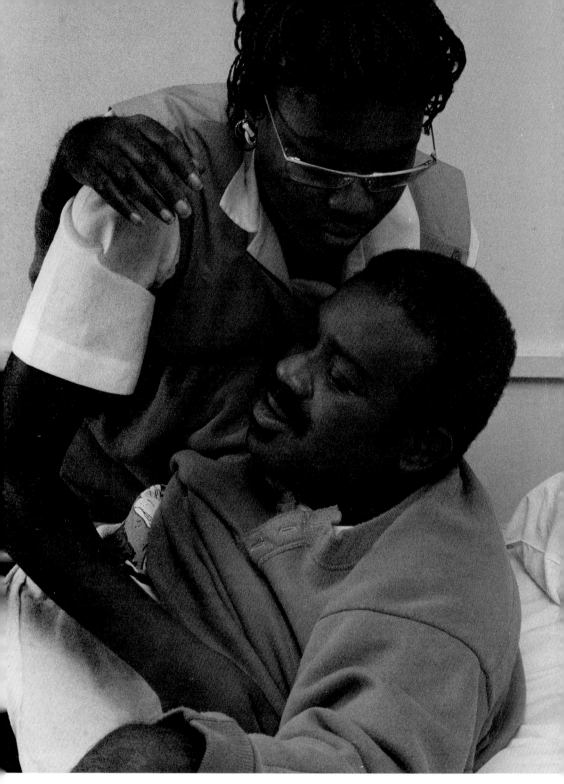

A career in health care gives you the opportunity to help others.

CAREERS & OPPORTUNITIES

CAREERS INSIDE THE WORLD OF
Health Care

by Beth Wilkinson

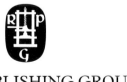

THE ROSEN PUBLISHING GROUP, INC.
NEW YORK

Published in 1995, 1999 by The Rosen Publishing Group, Inc.
29 East 21st Street, New York, New York 10010

Revised Edition 1999

Library of Congress Cataloging-in-Publication Data

Wilkinson, Beth.
    Careers inside the world of health care / by Beth Wilkinson.—
Rev. ed.
        p.   cm.   —   (Careers & opportunities)
    Includes bibliographical references and index.
    ISBN 0-8239-2886-1
    1. Medicine—Vocational guidance—Juvenile literature.
[1. Medical care—Vocational guidance. 2. Allied health care—
Vocational guidance. 3. Vocational guidance.]   I. Title.
II.Series.
    R690.W547   1999
    362.1'023'73   95-23177
                                                         CIP
                                                          AC

Contents

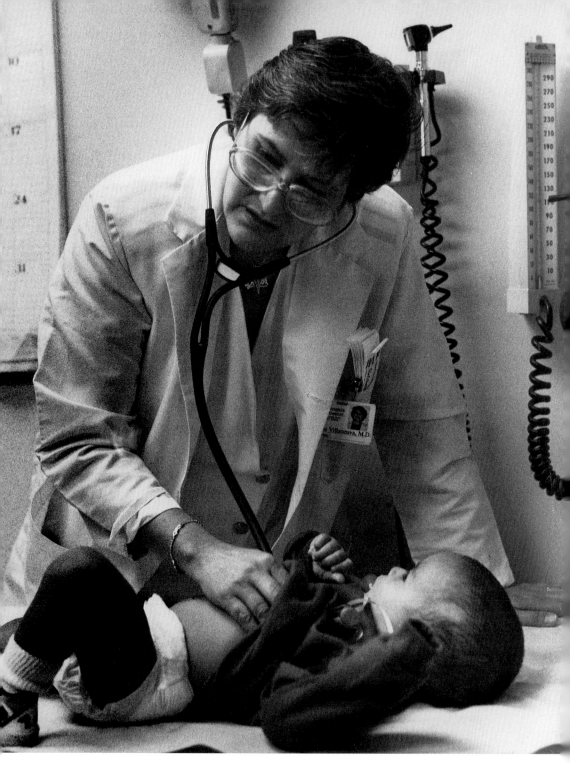

More than ever before in history, there is a great need for people in the field of health care.

CHAPTER 1

HEALTH CARE AS A CAREER

Are you curious about science? Do you enjoy doing experiments? Are articles, movies, or videos about medical technology fascinating to you? If so, such interest may indicate an inborn ability for a career in the growing field of health care. Another indication that you may be a natural for such a career is that the sight of blood doesn't upset you, and seeing excrement and other body wastes has never been a turn-off. Maybe wounds and punctures don't make you feel squeamish. In an emergency, you may have learned, you feel a need to rush to the rescue.

When you witness pain in others or other things, it may trigger compassion within you—and curiosity. When Lorenzo was ten years old he found a bird with a broken wing. "I felt terrible about the little creature's distress," he says, "but my main thought was how to fix the wing and get the bird flying again. In spite of a bird's

7

delicate nervous system and its almost certain death, the bird survived. That was when I knew that I was good at fixing hurts. It was the beginning of my journey into the medical field."

Like Lorenzo, you may be aware that you have certain gifts necessary to heal. Skills are required for working with the sick and infirm. So are compassion and tolerance. Anyone in health care must also be physically fit; the nature of the job often requires a person to lift, move, and shift patients. Your foremost traits may be a good attitude toward life and a desire to help others. Job descriptions and qualifications may differ, but all health care employment involves one basic requirement: you must like working with and caring for the sick and keeping them as physically healthy as possible.

Rewards

Flexible working hours, fringe benefits, and a pleasant atmosphere are some of the advantages of working in the health care community. Another big plus is that the men and women that you work with will have similar experiences, interests, and goals. Contributing to the wellness of others is not only satisfying, it is also profitable. In the health care occupations, salaries range from minimum wage in entry-level jobs to mega-dollar salaries earned by medical specialists.

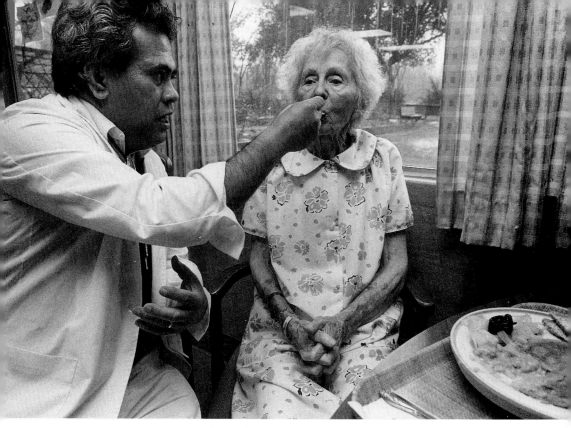
People are living longer because of better health care.

Job Possibilities

There is a demand for all kinds of professional
and semiprofessional workers in the medical field.
A wide range of highly respected jobs exist in the
health care industry. Many types of medical doctors,
such as oncologists, opthalmologists, pediatricians,
dermatologists, and radiologists, work in hospitals,
private offices, and clinics. These workplaces also
employ support personnel, such as secretaries,
clerks, and accountants. Nurses, too, work in
specialized fields such as emergency care, surgery,
and extended care units. Many people specialize in

9

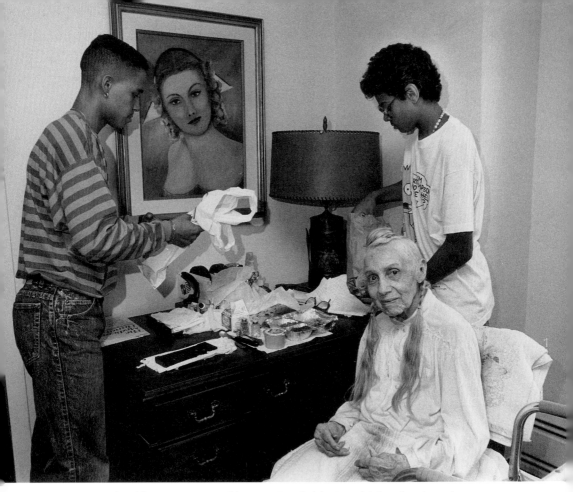

Home health care is a quickly growing field. Two high school students help an elderly woman get her dinner ready. Her arthritis makes it difficult to open the containers of food, so they do it for her.

rehabilitation services, such as physical therapy and speech pathology. Hospitals, private medical offices, and clinics need workers for laundry and janitorial crews. Food must be made available for patients in a hospital and for the patient's visitors, so dietitians, food servers, and kitchen help are always needed. Most hospitals need workers in the pharmacy, medical library, and gift shop.

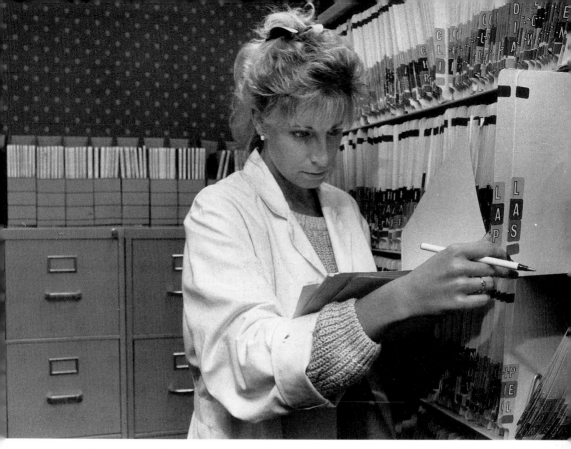

A visit to a physician's assistant is usually faster and less expensive than a visit to a doctor.

Other Pursuits

Dentistry has changed a great deal in recent years and requires people with different talents, knowledge, and visions. Look at movies, videos, and television shows and notice the actors' dazzling and perfect teeth. This is the result of a new and costly type of dentistry in which a dentist can bond, cap, and replace teeth. Even tooth transplants are possible. Incomes in this field exceed the $100,000 per year bracket. Dentists also employ assistants to prepare patients for treatment and hygienists to check and clean teeth.

Other important health care workers include pharmacists, and ambulance drivers and paramedics for emergencies and transportation of patients. Many careers are connected with bone and joint clinics and hospices (homelike facilities that provide care for the terminally ill). Midwives are becoming more popular, and there is an increasing demand for massage therapists.

Progress

Today, people are living decades longer. The life expectancy for men is 76, and for women it is 85. And with long life spans come different illnesses, aches, and pains.

In the 19th and early 20th centuries, certain illnesses and disorders, such as Alzheimer's disease, were unknown because people didn't live as long. Identified in the early 1900s by German physician Alois Alzheimer, Alzheimer's has only recently been acknowledged as one of the foremost medical problems of the elderly. In earlier times Alzheimer's was considered a form of dementia and was usually just accepted as a part of the aging process. There is no cure for this disease, but delaying the onset of the illness for even a few years will make a difference in the diagnosis, care, and span of the victim's life.

With scientific advances and new technology,

health care has become sophisticated. More people are able to live longer and enjoy their lives as healthy human beings. Twice as many drugs for managing the symptoms of diseases are available now as even a decade ago, and more are being discovered. The fact the people are living longer has led to the relatively new concept of home health care.

Home Health Care

Home health care helps the ill and elderly remain at home and live independently. Home health caseworkers help clients with household chores, showers, meal preparation, and even grocery shopping. Men and women called dispatchers and transporters provide transportation for those unable to drive to the doctor's or dentist's office, hospital, or pharmacy. There are personnel training programs available for this kind of work.

Many Possibilities

Many opportunities exist for young people in the field of medical research. In recent years important research has included the identification of HIV (human immunodeficiency virus), which causes the fatal sexually transmitted disease AIDS. Although no cure has been found, a longer life span for victims is now possible.

Popular interest in alternative medicine and

treatments such as homeopathy and stress management is on the rise. Pulmonary care, which provides oxygen for breathing illnesses, is a gratifying occupation that requires skilled workers.

Spin-off positions in health care include trainers at spas; managers of health food stores; and park and recreational directors. Office help is always needed in clinics and hospitals. Many of these jobs require a high school diploma or GED; some need a college degree.

The health care picture in the United States is constantly changing. This is evident from the increase in the number health maintenance organizations (HMOs); legislative proposals for a nationwide health care system; and changes in government sponsored programs such as Medicare. As successful treatments for more illnesses are discovered and health care reaches more people, the need for skilled medical workers in all fields will increase.

Questions to Ask Yourself

If you are considering a job in health care, there are many factors for you to consider, including the following: 1) Do you like being with different types of people? 2) Can you be sympathetic and patient with the sick and infirm? 3) Are you interested in the medical field?

CHAPTER 2

EXPERIENCE COUNTS

An entry-level job at a health care center will give you needed experience and could be your ticket to a lifelong career. Health care centers include hospitals, nursing homes, clinics, and private practices. Jobs in this field are listed in the classified section of most newspapers. Various positions, some requiring high school diplomas or college degrees, are usually found under the heading of "Help Wanted— Health/Medical." Salaries are often listed along with benefits, such as flexible hours and chances for advancement.

Other ads are aimed at those seeking training for health care careers. A sample ad reads: "Certified Nurse's Assistant Training Course. Share your love for caring. Prepare for the state examination. Small tuition fee." Usually these classes are held at a hospital, a civic center, or a

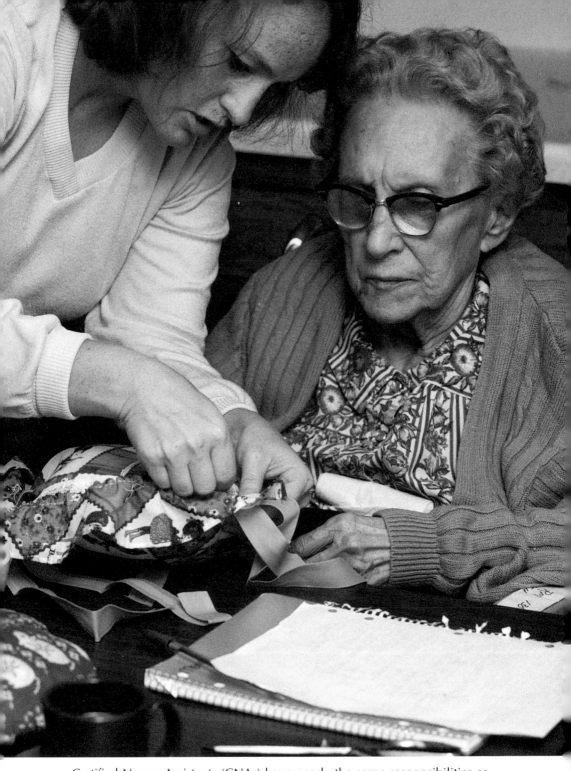

Certified Nurses Assistants (CNAs) have nearly the same responsibilities as Registered Nurses (RNs).

local school. They are taught by a nurse or a
certified nurse's assistant.

Clients and Convalescents

People who are cared for in nursing homes are of
all ages and have varying levels of disability. For
some clients, a mild memory loss may result in
failure to eat meals or take prescribed medication
regularly. Others have had strokes and are bed-
ridden. Some people suffer from respiratory diseases or debilitating conditions.

Carene

*Carene's grandmother, grandfather, and several
aunts are in their eighties and nineties. "Maybe
that's why I chose geriatrics [medical care for the
elderly] for a career," she says. "I've always related
to and enjoyed the elderly." After graduating from
high school Carene applied for and received a Pell
grant (which is based on financial need) and was
awarded a small academic scholarship by a professional women's group. It took her two years to earn
an associate degree in nursing. "I considered going on
for a bachelor of science in nursing (BSN), but getting that degree would take two additional years of
schooling, and there's not that much difference in
responsibilities or salary."*

Carene has definite ideas about how anyone

considering health care as a career should approach his or her education. "Before deciding on a lifetime of work in health care, learn as much as possible about it," she says. "Talk to doctors, nurses, and anyone who works in the field. Visiting a hospice or nursing home to talk with clients is a good start. You will be welcome. By observation, you'll learn simple things, like how to make a patient more comfortable in his or her bed, the importance of drinking liquids, and how to offer food to someone who can't feed himself. If you know some of these skills before entering a nursing program, you'll feel more confident.

"So enroll in any nursing class offered at your high school or junior college. Keep in touch with what is going on in the health industry by reading magazine and newspaper articles about newly discovered medical techniques and drugs. Television often presents information about health. Purchase a medical dictionary to become acquainted with the vocabulary of the field. Learn the different names of health care departments. You'll feel more secure if you know that the intensive care unit is called ICU (or critical care unit, CCU); the emergency room is called ER; obstetrics, OB; and the children's department is referred to as GYN/PD or Peds (pronounced "peeds"). When you're in a drug area of the supermarket, look at the shelves that hold over-the-counter remedies." Carene says it's a big

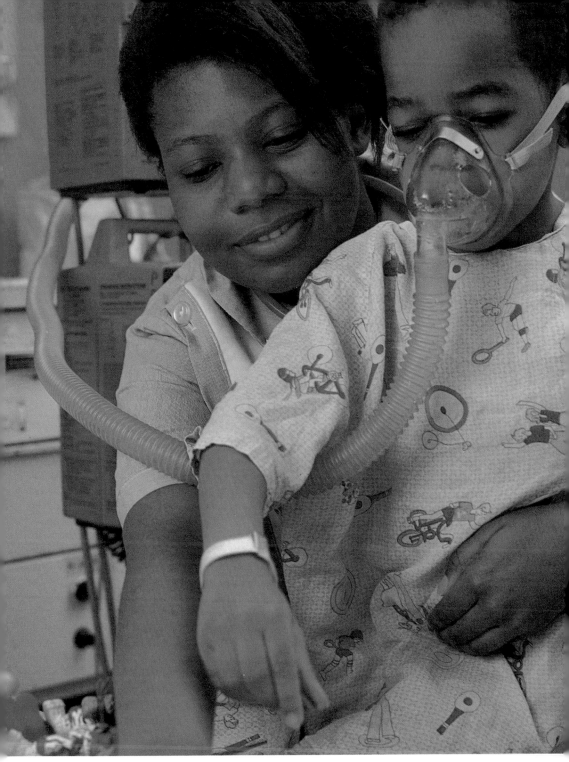

As a Certified Nurse's Assistant or a Registered Nurse you can work in many different departments. This nurse works in Pediatrics.

plus to work in a nursing home or care center. "It's wonderful to be able to take advantage of the wisdom and knowledge older people are willing to share."

Indeed, there are numerous pluses to working in the health care field. But as in all fields, there are also minuses. Night-shift work is often assigned to new employees. Dealing with dying patients can be difficult. It is easy for some people to become depressed because of the nature of the work; it requires special coping skills. Back trouble is also a common complaint. In fact, only employees in manual labor have more back problems than health care personnel.

Housekeeping and Environmental

Bud is employed in the same nursing home as Carene. He has been there for three years. He says he learned the work ethic from his mother, an Oglala Sioux, and his father, who emigrated from Northern Ireland. "I found my niche in maintenance," he says.

There it's his job to sweep, mop, strip, wax, and buff the linoleum floors of the halls, dining areas, and lounge, and to clean up the major spills in the patients rooms. "I mop boards and edgings with soap and hot water," he says. "I wipe down walls. On weekends I use an automatic scrubber with disinfectant and clean all floors."

For Bud, working at the center is a part-time job.

"I work from 8:00 PM to 10:00 PM five nights a week. Saturday and Sunday I work from 7:00 AM to 3:00 PM, then come back from 7:00 PM until 9:30 PM. I work 7 days a week. My job title is floor maintenance. I also have a full-time job at the high school, where I am listed as custodial maintenance engineer. My salary at the nursing home started at $3.75 an hour. Now I make $6.28 per hour, plus vacations and sick leave. Insurance covers dental care and hospitalization. For me, this place has the feeling of home. I even have a young relative working here. I never miss work because I'm never sick."

Broughan

Bud's cousin Broughan works in the nursing home's laundry, where the wearing of rubber gloves and an apron is a requirement for infection control. He likes the simple but important procedure of washing, drying, and folding sheets, pillowcases, towels, and the residents' personal clothing.

"A job in a laundry is the perfect place for me," Broughan says. *"I'm a student, and it gives me time to think about the night classes I'm enrolled in at the junior college. My work schedule is more or less flexible. For some reason the odors, which can sometimes be overwhelming in an institution, don't bother me. My long-term goal is to go into business, where the pay can be terrific, and maybe own or*

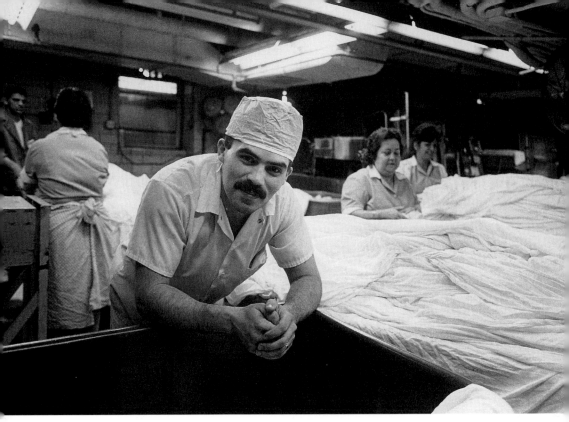

There are many ways to get involved in the field of health care. One way is through working in a laundry facility.

become administrator of a care center. Any kind of management entails paperwork, buying supplies, directing crews, making schedules, and promoting, hiring, and firing employees. Even though I do these things only on a small scale, I'm getting experience. I've found out that a good nursing home doesn't 'warehouse' the elderly; it offers many types of rehabilitation, such as physical, occupational, speech, and respiratory therapies. A guy that had been here for two years was recently released because, with therapy, he learned to get around."

22   Carene, Bud, and Broughan recommend that

young people interested in careers in health care get all the hands-on experience possible. This is sound advice from three people with solid backgrounds in the field.

Advancement, Growth and Headway

In recent years nursing homes have become a bridge between hospitals and patients' homes by providing rehabilitation services. A physical injury, disease, disability, or functional loss make it difficult to carry out everyday activities that most people take for granted.

For instance, crash victims discharged from the hospital need therapy to return to living independently. For these people, skills such as using a knife and fork or buttoning a shirt must be relearned. With therapy, patients relearn daily living skills such as eating, dressing, bathing, personal care, and homemaking. They are often able to return to a normal routine.

Nursing homes are no longer "the last stop."

Questions to Ask Yourself

Experience is a must for anyone interested in pursuing a career in health care. Ask yourself these questions: 1) What field of health care are you interested in? 2) How much schooling does this field require? 3) What is the best way for you to get experience in this field?

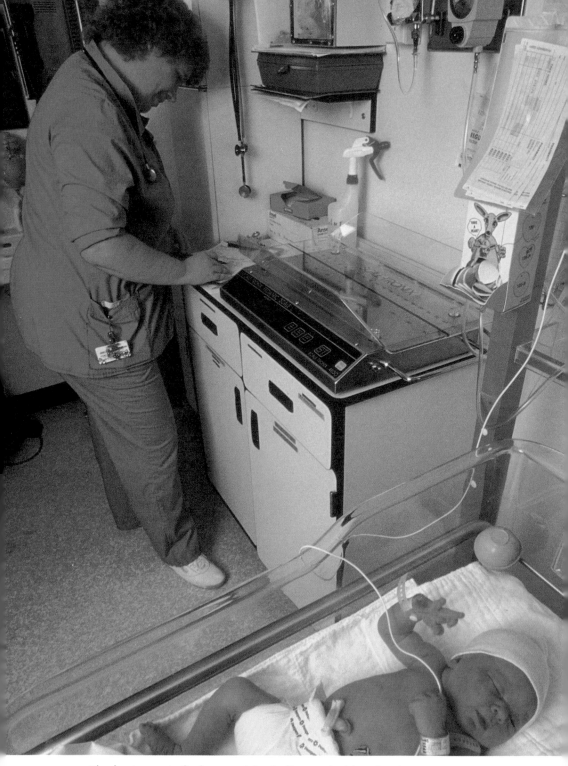

The best way to find your niche is first to decide what interests you.
This woman probably likes working with infants.

CHAPTER 3

A PLACE IN THE PICTURE

Health care careers are no longer gender-based. Men and women are equally encouraged to enter all levels of the medical profession. With additional education a person can advance in the medical field to jobs with better pay, larger benefits, and a more comfortable lifestyle. For some people the cost of advanced education—in interest, time, and money—is too high. Others find the pursuit a challenge. When it was suggested that a career as a surgeon took great commitment on his part, Dr. Etienne Bennett answered, "That's what I enjoy: being responsible for the improvement and recovery of patients' health. I also like being in charge."

Making Plans

In high school, Dustin considered science and biology his best subjects. Like Dr. Bennett, Dustin wanted to help alleviate pain and cure the sick. When Dustin's grandmother died of cancer, he decided to go to college and eventually go into cancer research as a biochemist. But things don't always work out the way they are planned, and Dustin has had to give up this idea for the time being. "Someday," he says, "I'll go into research. I'm saving money toward that goal."

Dustin's Story

"After high school, going on to university was out of the question because my parents got a divorce. I had to get a job and find my own place to live. I lucked out and was hired as a night maintenance man at the hospital. It felt good working there. During emergencies I was glad to help with uncooperative patients, usually people having drug reactions. I became interested in the emergencies and the ambulance drivers handled, and I asked about a job. I found out that there's a lot more to it than just learning to drive the ambulance. The bottom line is that I trained four months to be an Emergency Medical Technician (EMT). I was taught the signs and symptoms of drug overdose, diabetic coma, diseases, heart and asthma attacks, chronic bronchitis, and emphysema. I learned to administer IV's to replace body fluid in cases of trauma. I'm now able to treat shock and extricate accident victims from cars. I know how to use the backboard to stabilize the body, a cervical collar to protect the neck, and splints to

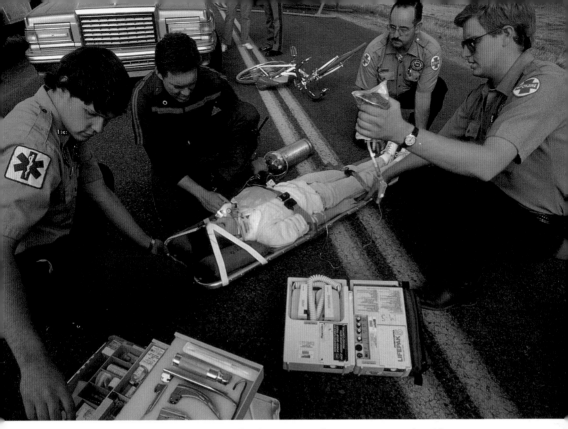

Paramedics play a vital role in providing emergency health care.

maintain the position of the limbs. In fact, an ambulance is a traveling emergency room."

Some of the requirements for this job are a high school diploma and a Class C driver's license. Salaries begin around $24,000 and with continuing education go to $32,000. An EMT also takes a course called ACLS: Avoidance Cardiac Life Support. He or she learns to identify irregular heartbeats and restore the heart's normal rhythm. A medical technician often makes split-second life-or-death decisions, and administers cardiac medication and oxygen.

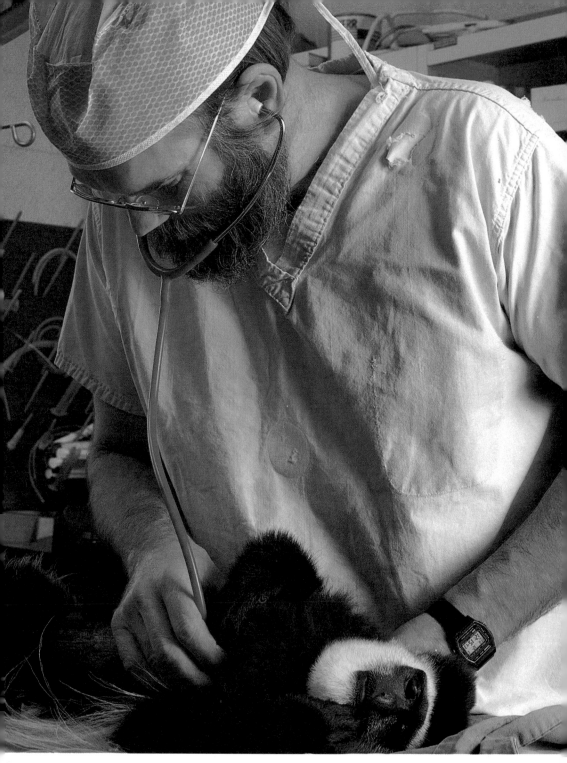

If you like animals you might want to consider a career in veterinary medicine.

Continued Training

Dustin is involved in ongoing education. "We keep up on the latest techniques for emergency health care and how we can best work with patients who attempt suicide or have seizures. Also, broken hips in senior citizens are not uncommon, and many emergency calls are from people who have fallen and been injured."

Men and women working as EMTs also take mental health classes to help reduce stress, Dustin says. "The nightmare calls for an ambulance driver or med tech are when children are involved: child abuse, or an injury that could have been prevented if the child had been in a car seat or wearing a seatbelt. Fortunately, my mind is so full of what has to be done that I often don't notice all the blood. The important thing is to get to the hospital."

The Introduction

Lorenzo says that as long as he can remember he has loved being around animals. When he was a child, dogs, cats, birds, rabbits, and tanks of fish were an important part of the family. Lorenzo didn't mind doing his share of feeding and watering these creatures. At his grandparents' farm he spent as much time as possible in the barns. His grandfather, thinking he was encouraging a future farmer, taught his grandson how to milk a cow, feed the chickens,

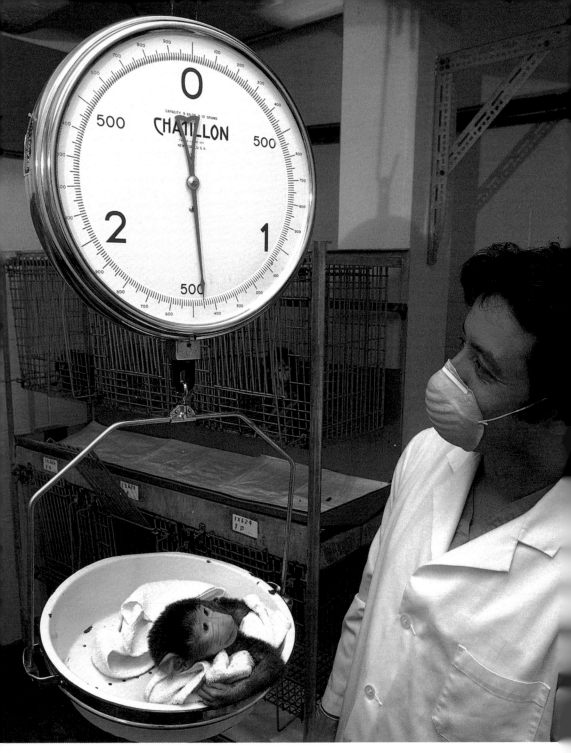

One way to get into veterinary medicine is to begin as an animal attendant. With training you can become an Animal Health Technician (AHT).

and gather eggs. As Lorenzo grew, he learned how to clean stalls and replenish nesting sites. In the spring he watched lambs being born and learned to pull calves when the need came up. While his grandfather dreamed of his grandson becoming a farmer and taking over the farm, Lorenzo dreamed of being able to work with animals and healing them.

The Dream Goes On

Lorenzo's first job was as an animal attendant at a veterinary clinic. His job was to clean cages and feed and water the animals. "It was a piece of cake," he says. I learned to do things like that at the farm before I could walk." For this he was paid minimum wage. His first goal was to enter a college-level program to become an Animal Health Technician (AHT). The job, with a starting salary of $7.00 per hour, was working in an animal clinic. Some states, including the one Lorenzo lived in, require licensing, which means that certain requirements must be met and an examination passed. "As an AHT my duties included preparing the animals and instruments for surgery, and giving medication," Lorenzo says. Lorenzo's grandfather was disappointed that his grandson would not someday take over the family farm. "Nevertheless," Lorenzo says, "he encouraged me in my career choice, and I completed my course work in a year and two summers."

Another Big Decision

A few years later Lorenzo's grandfather died and his grandmother moved into a retirement center. The farm was sold. When Lorenzo shared his dream of being a veterinarian with his grandmother, she did not hesitate to say that she wanted to help him through school. "Your grandfather would approve," she told her grandson. Lorenzo completed his undergraduate study and then finished four years of veterinary school.

A veterinarian may work with birds, fish, reptiles, or domestic, exotic, or farm animals. A doctor of veterinary medicine (D.V.M.) may care for small or large animals or specialize in fields such as surgery, acupuncture, or opthalmology (eye care). As for a medical doctor, the salary depends on area of specialization, the hours he or she puts in, and whether the person is the employer or is employed by someone else.

Alternate Plans

No one can predict what the future holds. Unforeseen events can interfere with plans and expectations of life. As time passes, a person may discover a more interesting career path to follow. Therefore people need to have alternate goals as backups for their original career plans. The health care field certainly provides a multitude of choices.

CHAPTER 4

AN OVERVIEW

An important part of having good health is to care for one's physical, mental, and social well-being. It is this feeling of well-being that sets the tone for all of us, from birth to death. That is why taking care of ourselves is so important. Among recommendations to meet this goal are annual physical examinations by a physician, regular visits to the dentist, and routine appointments with an ophthalmologist or optometrist for eye checkups. Often, hearing tests by an audiologist are essential for maintaining a healthy lifestyle. It is vital that people take the initiative in being responsible for their good health. Nowadays, more and more patients are taking charge of their health and their lives.

Science

The saying "You've come a long way, baby" applies to the field of medical research. Some technology used only a few years ago has been replaced with newer and more successful procedures. For example, doctors have discovered a new technique to halt the devastation that Parkinson's disease brings to some 1.5 million Americans. A spectacular success story, reported in the *Denver Post,* tells about Karen Stephani, a casualty of this crippling neurological condition. After trying an experimental brain implant, she is now regaining her strength well enough to put away her wheelchair. "I was instantly better," said Stephani four months after surgeons drilled a hole in her skull and implanted a device that essentially blocked the motor-control symptoms of Parkinson's disease. "I don't want to be gushy, but it's very exciting," said Dr. Mark Stacy, director of the Muhammad Ali Parkinson's Research Center in Phoenix, who advises the National Parkinson Foundation. While this disease has not yet been cured, the symptoms can be suppressed.

These are exciting times in which to enter the field of health care. Many different health care jobs exist. The following is a brief list of some options.

Dental Caretakers

Prominent among health care providers are dentists, dental assistants, and hygienists. Different dental offices will have other employees

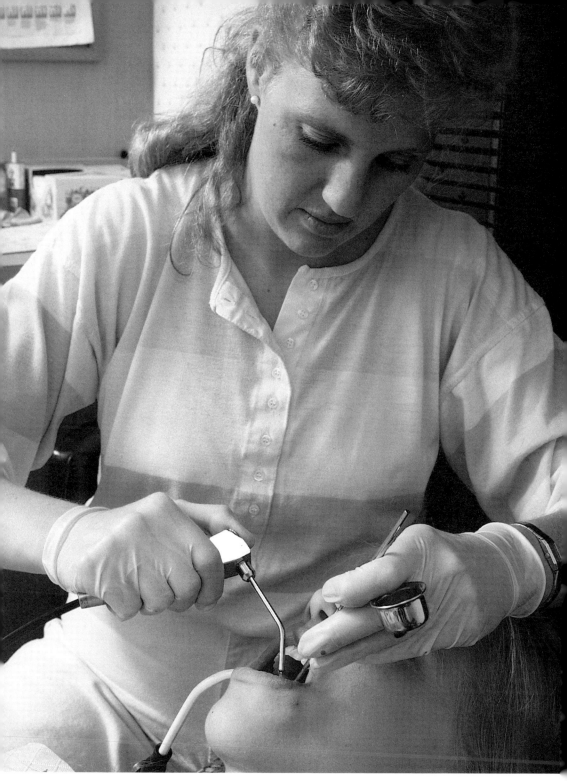

Dental caretakers are important in the field of health.

with various skills, but this is the general organization of a dental office.

Dentist's Office

The staff of Dr. Becki Burman's dental office consists of four people: Becki, who has been a practicing dentist for five years; Faun, the receptionist; Gaylene, the dental assistant; and Nancy, the dental hygienist. The situation is ideal for these young women. They are all mothers and can take their babies to work. A room has been set aside as a nursery, and a sitter is provided. Each of these women started out in a dental office as a receptionist or dental assistant. Depending on state laws, those jobs do not always require more than a high school education.

Several years ago, during school vacation, Nancy worked as a dental assistant for her father. "As a dental assistant, I didn't have to go to a university," Nancy says, "but I did go to nine weeks of X-ray school to earn a registered dental assistant certificate." Nancy found the work interesting. "Mixing the silver for a filling after the dentist had prepared the tooth was one of my duties. I liked the responsibility of ordering the dental supplies, too. I met a lot of neat people, and I considered the job a lot of fun. A couple of years later I decided to be a dental hygienist, because I had had a son, and I needed a bigger salary. I enrolled in a two-year course at a community college.

It wasn't easy, but I earned an associate degree in applied science (dental hygiene) and passed a required state test. Right now my ongoing education consists of attending hygienists' conferences and workshops twice a year."

Recently Nancy took a short course on administrating local anesthetics. She also enrolled in a workshop to learn about tooth extractions, restorative dental care, and the technique of removing deep scale tartar from fillings. Nancy also has plans for the future. "I think that some day, when my baby is older, I may go to dental school and become a dentist. Of course, that's far in the future, but because of my background as an assistant and a hygienist, the prospect is there. In dentistry a person with determination can continue improving his or her career because the jobs are layered: receptionist, dental assistant, dental hygienist, and of course, the dentist. In this job if you are willing to work hard you can go as high on the salary scale as you desire. An average hourly wage for my job is $18.50."

Audiologist

An audiologist's job is to identify, chart, diagnose, treat, and work to prevent hearing problems. He or she also tests hearing, usually with an audiometer, which measures sound at various frequencies. When a hearing loss is found, a course of action is recommended. It may be the removal of ear wax, the use of a hearing aid, or surgery.

Audiologists may work, in a clinic, a hospital, or in private practice. Public school systems employ audiologists to test children's hearing; such employment requires a graduate college degree. As people age, their hearing worsens. Because the average American is getting older, the need for specialists in this field is tremendous. The range of salaries is $26,000 to $42,000 per year.

Therapist

Therapists, also called allied health personnel, are important in today's world of life in the fast lane. Physical therapists are trained to treat or help rehabilitate people who have been ill or injured. They help patients relearn the tasks of everyday living. Their methods include exercise, heat treatments, and massage. Speech therapists identify speech disabilities and help overcome them by use of tongue exercises and speech drills. They are able to teach a patient to speak and swallow. Psychologists practice another type of therapy. They use psychological methods for rehabilitation of the sick or wounded or in helping people overcome emotional problems. Therapists find employment in hospitals, rehabilitation centers, clinics, public schools, or

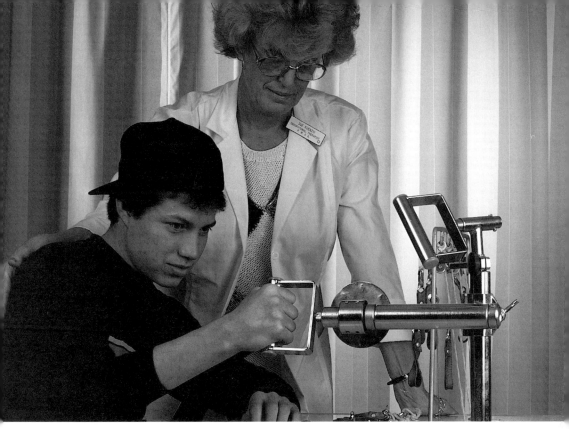
Physical therapists are trained to help rehabilitate people who have been ill or injured.

private practice. Educational requirements vary considerably. Salaries, depending on expertise, range from $25,348 up.

Ophthalmologists and Optometrists

More than half of Americans wear contact lenses or eyeglasses. Ophthalmologists are physicians who specialize in diagnosis and treatment of eye diseases and injuries. They also do eye surgery and prescribe corrective lenses. Their education is comparable to that of other medical doctors, with corresponding salaries.

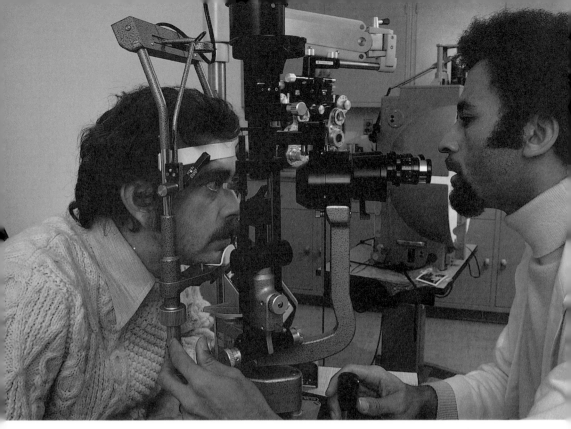

There are several areas within the field of eye care. Ophthalmology and optometry are just two.

Optometrists provide most of the primary vision care needed by people over 45. At least two or three years of pre-optometry study at a college or university are required before entering a four-year course at an optometry school. Most optometrists earn a bachelor's degree before entering optometry school. Salaries start at about $65,000 per year.

A dispensing optician is a person who helps clients select frames and fits and adjusts glasses. A laboratory technician makes prescription glasses. Salaries in these areas range from $15,000 to $25,000 per year.

"Nurse Calling"

More and more patients are taking control of their lives. They gather facts about their health from many sources. With information concerning health issues, men and women are often able to prolong their lives. In some states a special telephone number is maintained for people needing answers to simple health questions. This service may be called Nurse Calling or Health Answers. The person answering the telephone is a registered nurse. Using a computer, the nurse can find up to 350 formal answers, known as protocols, to health questions and can consult a library for other requested information. These people do not diagnose illness, which cannot be done by phone. But they do provide a helpful service for the public.

Questions to Ask Yourself

The careers in the health care world are many and varied. Here are some questions that might help you decide which is best for you. 1) Do you prefer to work with people, or behind the scenes? 2)Do you prefer a structured schedule, or would you like to be on call? 3) Would you prefer to work with the young, the elderly, or those in between?

CHAPTER 5

SPECIAL CARE

Working in the field of health care offers advantages such as flexible hours, steady income, and a pleasant atmosphere. Beginning salaries appear to be improving. In addition, fringe benefits increase employees' yearly earnings. Some of these benefits may include health and dental insurance, life insurance, and retirement plans. According to a 1996 *U.S. News and World Report* survey, the average salaries in specialized health care at the entry level are $24,000, midlevel, $36,000 and top, $64,000. These are some things you might want to think about when considering a career in health care.

Licensed Practical Nurse

LPNs care for the physically and mentally ill, newborns, and the aged, and assist registered nurses and doctors. A high school diploma or a GED is necessary to be accepted into a one- to

two-year training program. A written examination
is required in all states before a person can be
licensed. LPNs' earnings range from about
$25,000 per year up to a top salary of $30,000 to
$35,000 per year.

Midwife

Midwives support women during pregnancy,
assist the mother during labor and delivery, and
provide prenatal and postnatal care. Midwives
may be trained through apprenticeship, or they
may be certified nurse midwives—registered
nurses who have completed one to two years of
extra training in an accredited midwifery program.
Fees range from $900 to $1,500 per assignment.

Registered Nurse

RNs care for the injured and ill. They assist
physicians and surgeons with patient examinations
and operations. They can also teach, work as
private-duty nurses, or work in businesses,
private homes, schools, clinics, or physicians'
offices. Requirements are a high school
education, two to four years in nursing school,
and passing of a licensing examination. Many
nursing programs are available. Salaries vary
depending on location and training, but the
average salary is $43,181 per year and rising.

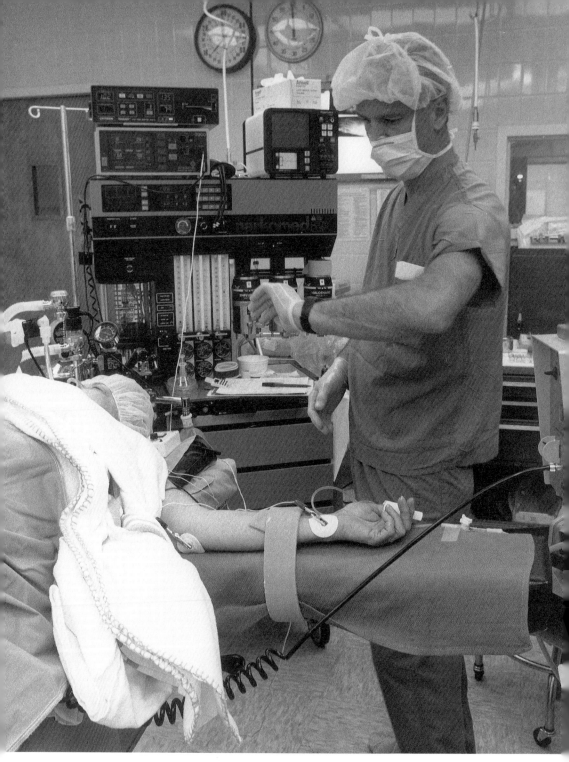

Nurse anesthetists administer drugs to induce sleep, deaden pain, or help patients relax during surgery.

Nurse Anesthetist

These technicians administer drugs to induce sleep, help deaden pain, or allow patients to relax during surgery. They work in operating, delivery, and emergency rooms. Nurse anesthetists must first become registered nurses and then take a one- to two-year special training program. Practicing nurse anesthetists must be licensed. The median annual base salary for full-time nurse anesthetists is $82,000.

Nurse Practitioner

Nurse practitioners are registered nurses who have completed additional two- to four-year certification programs. They are able to determine causes of illnesses and plan appropriate treatment. They offer preventive medical services and provide long-term care for a variety of health problems. In many states, nurse practitioners can also prescribe medication. Their salaries may be double those of registered nurses.

Nursing and Psychiatric Aide

This work entails the care of people who are physically or mentally ill. Basic duties include serving meals; answering patients' call bells; taking temperatures; and undressing, bathing, and dressing patients. A high school diploma or GED is preferred. Hospitals and nursing homes offer on-the-job training and ongoing education. According to a University of Texas survey, the weekly earnings of full-time salaried nursing and psychiatric aides were $274 to $482.

X-ray Technologist

Working with radiologists, these specialists diagnose and treat diseases using x-ray and radioactive material. A high school diploma is required to enroll in a two- or four-year radiographic technology program offered by hospitals, medical schools, and universities. The salary range for this position is $10.18 per hour minimum to $19.20 per hour maximum.

Making Choices

People who care for the ill make an important and necessary contribution to society. However, not everyone has the aptitude or the desire to work with suffering and even dying men, women, and children. When considering your life's work, you would be wise to evaluate your interests and personal qualities. If working directly with sick people, waste, or blood products would be difficult for you, the following options may be of interest to you.

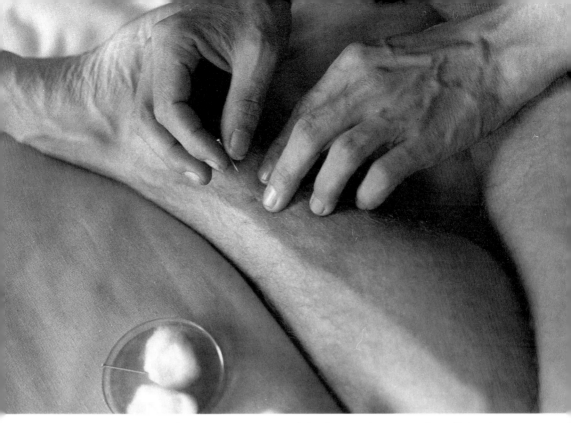

Acupuncture is becoming a more widely accepted system of medicine in the West.

Acupuncturist

Acupuncture is a system of medicine that has been used in China for more than 5000 years. The acupuncturist uses needles to treat injury, pain, and illness, and to prevent sickness. Persons wanting to enter this profession need at least two years of college and three years of study at an accredited school or with an experienced acupuncturist. Salaries range widely, from moderate pay to as much as $100,000 per year.

Cardiovascular Technologists

These technicians work primarily in intensive

care units at hospitals, using computer equipment to evaluate patients' heartbeats. A two-year junior or community college program and on-the-job training are required. Average salaries are $20,200 to $25,000 per year.

Chiropractor

Chiropractors treat muscle and bone pain by manipulation and adjustment of the patient's body, especially the spine. This profession requires a high school diploma, two years of college, and four years at a chiropractic college. The salary range is $20,000 to $180,000.

Dietitian

Dietitians are experts in nutrition and food management. They plan menus and diets for people with special needs and work in hospitals, community centers, nursing homes, and schools. They are high school graduates, have degrees in dietetics, and take training programs in hospitals. Salaries range from $21,800 to $35,500.

Home Health Care Aide

This work involves the care and emotional support of the ill and assistance with household tasks. There are no specific educational requirements, although high school graduation is a plus. The pay is minimum wage to $8.00 per hour.

Homeopath

Homeopathy, which seeks to use natural substances to heal patients, is becoming a widespread form of health care. Practitioners use small doses of natural substances to stimulate a patient's immune and defense systems. Childhood diseases, infections, allergies, and chronic illnesses are some of the conditions addressed by homeopathy. Homeopaths are often physicians who are also trained in herbal medicine and nutrition. Income is comparable to that of conventionally trained doctors.

Hospital Administrator

Responsibilities involve supervision of staff, purchasing, use of building and equipment, preparation of budgets, and decisions on future needs. A master's degree is often required. The salary ranges from $90,000 at a small hospital to $225,000 in a large city medical center.

Medical Records Assistant

The major responsibilities are to assist professionals and to keep records. A high school diploma and graduation from a training program are needed. Part-time work is often possible, with salaries of about $7,000 to $15,000 per year.

Pharmaceutical Industry Worker

Work in this field is in factories that produce medicines. Workers mix substances operate machines to make tablets or capsules. A high school diploma or a GED is preferred. Average earnings are $21,000 per year.

Pharmacist

Pharmacists fill prescriptions written by doctors and dentists. They often are able to recommend medications to ease minor illnesses. A high school education, five years of pharmacy school, and a one-year internship under an accredited pharmacist are required, as is state licensing. Salaries range between $49,000 and $58,000 yearly and are rising.

Questions to Ask Yourself

Not all careers in health care require you to deal with blood. If you'd like to work in health care but don't have the stomach to work with body fluids, ask yourself these questions. 1) Are you good with numbers, relish reading and doing reports? 2) Are you willing to complete the required schooling for positions of high responsibility?

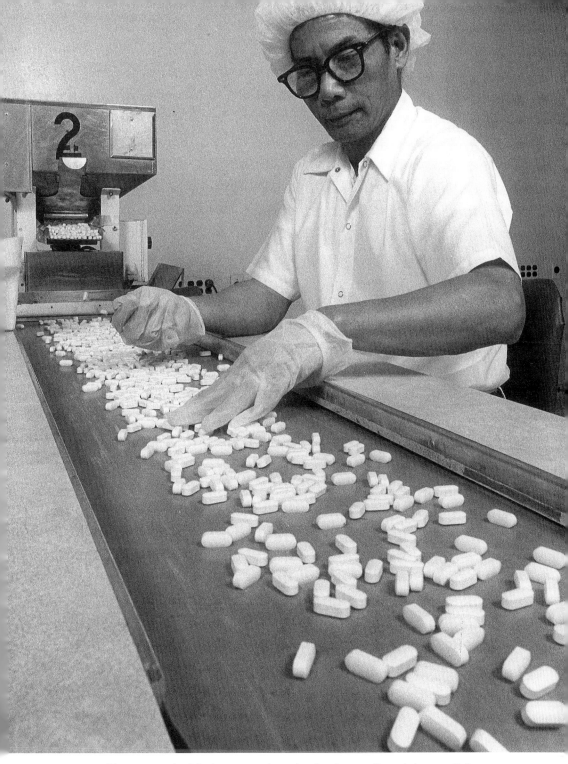

Pharmaceutical industry worker checks the quality of the medicine produced.

CHAPTER 6

WORKING UP THE JOB LADDER

The health care industry includes more of the best-paying and fastest-growing jobs for the twenty-first century than virtually any other job category. The increase is driven by new technology that keeps people alive longer, the AIDS epidemic, the aging population of America, and the growing importance of health care.

David

After school, David, age fifteen, had a part-time job at a popular Mexican restaurant. After graduating from high school he started working full-time at the same place. "I liked the food," he says.

A short stay as a patient at the hospital changed his mind about his earlier career choice. "I was impressed by the hospital workers' dedication. Even the food was good."

David started in an entry-level job and claims

that it was the best decision he's ever made. As a patient service associate (PSA), he was responsible for cleaning rooms, helping patients order meals, delivering trays, and charting what patients ate. PSAs do not touch or handle patients.

David worked in housekeeping for three months and then studied to become a certified nurse's aid (CNA). He worked in extended care for four months. Some of David's duties were to check blood pressure, help with bathing, and change dressings. Pivoting, lifting, and walking patients were among his duties.

Next, David opted to work on the surgery orthopedic floor as a CNA and unit secretary. His duties included entering the results of X rays and lab work into the computer; transcribing doctors' handwritten orders for nurses, and logging patients' vital statistics, surgery records, and length of hospital stay. Other responsibilities included ordering X rays and blood work and shaving patients in preparation for surgery.

After working for four years at the hospital, David is now a secretary medical/surgical technician (MST). This entails setting up interviews with patients and answering many questions about surgery. "A lot of social work is involved in this job," David says, "such as talking people through tough times. I am aware that part of my gift for working with sick people is gentleness and the ability to diffuse anger."

David's present goal is to become a surgical nurse,

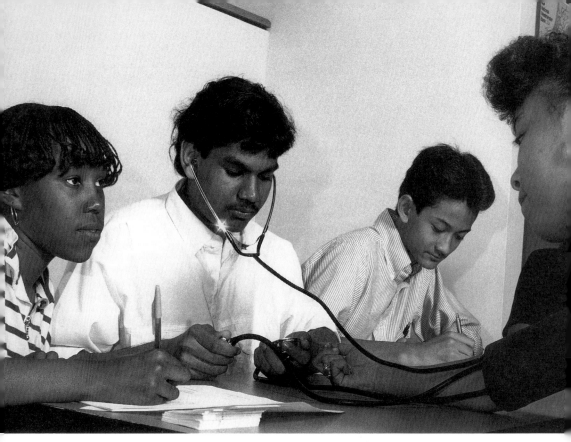

You might work as a summer intern through school to gain experience in the medical field. These students are learning how to check blood pressure.

which requires four years at a university. "It will take time, money, and energy," David says. In one corner of this young man's brain is a desire to become a doctor. "That was my ambition when I was a little kid," he says. "One thing I know is that I'm a service-oriented person. Health care, in any form, is the ultimate service-oriented post, and a hospital is a great place to work."

David may someday realize his dream of becoming a doctor. College courses in science are necessary for admittance to medical school. Study at medical school generally takes six to eight years, after which a student must fulfill at least three years of residency.

Physicians

Doctors are called specialists when they are experts in a particular area of medicine. There are many specialties in medicine. A general practitioner practices general medicine, performs some surgery, and delivers babies. An internist diagnoses and treats conditions affecting the internal organs of the body. The psychiatrist is also a medical doctor. After medical school, he or she must complete additional years of schooling before entering practice. Psychiatrists investigate the unconscious mental processes of a patient and treat mental and emotional problems. Endocrinologists specialize in treating the glands, such as the pituitary and thyroid. An allergist diagnoses and treats allergies, a pediatrician cares for children's health, and a geriatrician treats the elderly. These professionals are licensed by state and medical societies. Physicians have among the highest earnings of any occupation, often starting at $115,000 to $230,000 or more per year.

Making It Work For You

By the year 2000 a large population growth of men aged 76 and women 85 years old and above is expected. Workers of all kinds will be needed, not only for hospitals and nursing homes, but also for home health care, adult day-care programs, life-care communities, and assisted living arrangements. For these jobs a high school education is always preferred and is usually required for advancement, though sometimes a GED is acceptable. "Today low-entry hospital jobs are harder to come by than when I started years ago," David says. "If I were advising anyone on how to enter the health care field I would recommend taking health, science, math, botany, biology, chemistry, and computer courses. Applying at a nursing home is a good start. Also, being a volunteer at a health center is a good idea. It's rewarding, too."

Applying for a Job

When you wish to apply for a job, you will be more successful if you prepare yourself.

- Learn about the organization where you wish to work.
- Fill out a job application carefully; answer all questions.
- Practice an interview with a friend
- Arrive when your interview is scheduled.
- Be well-groomed and dress appropriately.
- Don't chew gum, smoke, or carry a soda
- Shake hands with your future employer.

- Use proper English.
- Relax and answer questions concisely.
- Listen to your interviewer.
- Thank the interviewer.

Other Job Tips
- Always carry your social security number and driver's license.
- Have a résumé of previous employment, education and training.
- Take references. Get permission to use names.

The Field Is Growing
Today there are many jobs in the field of health care that were unknown only a short time ago. Career opportunities have opened in designing special clothing and accessible furniture for people with disabilities. There is a demand for skilled workers at spas, gyms, and health food stores. Employment can also be found in pulmonary care: delivering oxygen to patients and providing respiratory therapy. Medical research is expanding, and medical library assistants are needed to catalog, file, and copy articles for physicians and staff. If you are serious about being a health care worker, you have a multitude of prospects to consider and pursue. If this is your dream, don't hesitate. You are needed.

GLOSSARY

acupuncture Chinese medical practice that endeavors to cure illnesses by puncturing specified areas of the body with needles.

AIDS (acquired immunodeficiency syndrome) A viral disease that weakens the immune system and leaves the body open to serious, often fatal infections.

Alzheimer's disease Brain disease that impairs mental and physical powers.

anesthetist Specially trained person who administers sedative drugs.

certified Having fulfilled legal requirements.

cervical Pertaining to the neck.

CNA Certified Nurse's Assistant

dedication Devotion and regard for a person, principle, career, or place.

dermatology Science of dealing with skin and its diseases.

facilities Building or office designed to offer special services.

GED Graduate Equivalency Program

hepatitis Inflammation of the liver.

homeopath One who treats diseases with small doses of herbs and drugs.

hospice Retreat or shelter for the terminally ill.

immune Exempt or protected from disease.

infection Contamination by disease-producing germs

laser Radiation device used in medicine.

midwife Woman who assists women in childbirth.

nutrition Food required for all living things to grow and develop.

ophthalmologist Doctor of medicine who treats diseases of the eyes.

paramedic Person skilled in emergency medical treatment.

Parkinson's disease Brain disease that affects mental and motor activity.

practitioner Person who specializes in mental health.

psychiatrist Doctor who specializes in mental health.

rehabilitation Treatment to restore either mental or physical health.

respiratory Pertaining to the body's breathing system.

technician Person trained for specialized work.

therapist Person trained to treat patients with specific mental or physical disorders.

volunteer Person who contributes services without payment.

APPENDIX

Volunteering at a hospital, nursing home, hospice, or school for the disabled is a good way to gain experience for working in health care. Most health care institutions have on-the-job programs to train those interested in such careers. Information about occupations requiring less than a year of preparation—such as dental assistant, medical assistant, or medical receptionist/secretary— is offered by Bryman School, 1144 West 3300 South, Salt Lake City, UT 84119-3330.

For details about other careers in health care, write to the following organizations:

American Association for Respiratory Care
11030 Ables Lane
Dallas, TX 75229
(972) 243-2272
http://www.aarc.org

American Association of Colleges of Nursing
One Dupont Circle NW, Suite 530
Washington, DC 20036
http://www.aacn.nche.edu

American Health Care Association
1201 L Street NW
Washington, DC 20005
http://www.ahca.org

American Hospital Association
Division of Health Careers
One North Franklin
Chicago, IL 60606
http://www.aha.org

American Occupational Therapy Association
1383 Piccard Drive
Rockville, MD 20850
http://www.aota.org

Canadian Institute for Health Information
377 Dalhousie Street, Suite 200
Ottawa, ON K1N 9N8
Canada
http://www.cihi.ca

Children's Hospice International
901 North Washington Street
Alexandria, VA 22314

**Jobs for Which You Can Train Through
 Apprenticeship**
U.S. Department of Labor
Bureau of Labor Statistics
Washington, DC 20212

National Council on Rehabilitation Education
1200 Commercial
Emporia State University
Emporia, KS 66801

National Association for Home Care
519 C Street NE
Washington, DC 20002

FOR FURTHER READING

Degens, T. *On the Third Ward.* New York: HarperCollins, 1990.

Exploring Health Care Careers, Vols. 1 and 2. Chicago: J. G. Fergusen Publishing Co., 1997.

Field, Shelly. *Career Opportunities in Health Care.* New York: Facts on File, 1997.

Gordon, Susan, and Hohenadel, Kristin. *Careers without College: Health Care.* Princeton, NJ: Peterson's, 1992.

Hayes, David, ed. *Exploring Health Care Careers: Real People Tell You What You Need to Know.* Chicago: Ferguson Publishing Co., 1997.

Lee, Barbara. *Working in Health Care and Wellness.* Minneapolis, MN: Lerner Publications Company, 1996.

Steinfeld, Alan. *Careers in Alternative Health Care.* New York: Rosen Publishing Group, 1996.

White, Ellen Emerson. *The Road Home.* New York: Scholastic, Inc., 1994.

INDEX

63

About the Author
Beth Wilkinson has been a career teacher for twenty-five years. Her goal has been to make lifetime readers out of students, friends, and family members. Hobbies and interests include arrowhead and potsherd hunting, collecting children's books, mountain hiking, viewing old movies, and writing poetry.

Cover Photo: © Barros and Barros/Image Bank
Photo Credits: pp. 2, 10, 54 © Ansell Horn/Impact Visuals; p. 6 © H. L Degado/Impact Visuals; p. 9 © Evan Johnson/Impact Visuals; p. 11 © Earl Dotter/Impact Visuals; p. 16 © Gary Bistram/Image Bank; p. 19 © Flip Chalfant/Image Bank; p. 22 © Penny Coleman/Impact Visuals; pp. 24, 27 © Anthony A. Boccaccio/Image Bank; p. 28 © Kay Chernush/Image Bank; p. 30 © David Vladimir Lance/Image Bank; p. 40 © Ira Block/Image Bank; p. 44 © Martha Tabor/Impact Visuals; p. 47 © Marty Heitner/Impact Visuals; p. 51 © Harvey Finkle/Impact Visuals
Photo Research: Vera Ahmedzadah
Design: Kim Sonsky